Navigating Grief

— With —

God

Finding Hope After Loss

By

NJ Domrufus

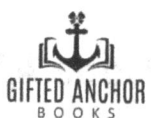

GIFTED ANCHOR
B O O K S

Gifted Anchor Books
ISBN: 9781965945247

Printed in the United States of America.

Dedication

To my dad, Mr. DomRufus Enemchukwu, whose love, strength, and gentle guidance shaped me into who I am today. Your memory lives on in every lesson and every cherished moment we shared.

And to Papa, Chief Christian Momah—You were a pillar of wisdom and warmth. Your kindness and unwavering support will always be remembered.

This book is for both of you, in honor of the love that never fades, even after loss.

Acknowledgements

Grief is a journey that connects us, and this book is the result of many voices, hearts, and hands that have walked alongside me. To my family, friends, church community, and all who have shared their stories—thank you for your unwavering love, support, and courage. Your strength and faith have inspired every word of this book. To the readers, thank you for trusting me to walk with you on your journey of loss and healing. And to God, thank you for being the source of all comfort and love. To my loving husband and two beautiful daughters—your support means everything to me.

With gratitude.

Dr. NJ Domrufus, DNP

Table of Contents

Forward

Grief is a journey we never plan for, yet it finds us all at some point in our lives. It comes uninvited, altering the rhythm of our days and leaving us to navigate a path we never wished to walk. In Navigating Grief with God: Finding Hope After Loss, Dr. NJ offers a lifeline to those who are struggling to make sense of their pain—a path through sorrow that is paved with faith, hope, and love.

As a mental health professional and a devoted believer, Dr. NJ brings a unique perspective to the journey of grieving. She knows what it means to sit in the quiet stillness of loss, to feel the questions and the heartache that accompany it. Her gentle guidance is not only rooted in her professional experience but also in her deep, personal understanding of God's love and grace.

This book is not about finding a way around grief but finding a way through it. Dr. NJ invites us to embrace our pain, to honor the love that lies beneath it, and to allow ourselves to be vulnerable in our grief. She reminds us that there is strength in our vulnerability, and that healing is possible—not because we are strong enough on our own, but because God walks with us every step of the way.

In the pages ahead, you will find practical tools for coping with loss, real-life stories that remind you that you are not alone, and reflections that speak directly to the heart of your pain. Dr. NJ's words are filled with compassion, wisdom, and the assurance that even in the darkest moments, God's presence is there, offering us hope.

Navigating Grief with God is a reminder that while grief may change us, it does not have to defeat us. It is an invitation to lean into God's comfort, to find strength in community, and to trust that there is light on the other side of sorrow. As you read these pages, may you find solace, may you find hope, and may you remember that even in the midst of your grief, you are deeply loved.

Okechukwu Nwachukwu

Authors Note

Dear Reader,

If you're holding this book, you may be walking through a season of loss or trying to support someone who is. Grief is a journey none of us ask for, yet it finds us all. The pain of losing someone dear can feel overwhelming, like waves that won't recede. And yet, in those waves, we find both the ache of absence and the tender traces of love that remain. It's a journey of heartbreak and transformation.

As a psychiatric mental health provider and a strong Christian, I've had the honor of walking with individuals and families through some of their most difficult moments. This book reflects both my professional insights and my deep faith in God's presence. In *Navigating Grief with God: Finding Hope After Loss*, my goal is not to provide a "solution" for grief—grief isn't something that needs solving. Instead, I hope to offer a companion for your journey. This book weaves together my experiences, stories of others who have walked this road, and the enduring comfort of Scripture. It's a guide to honoring our pain without letting it define us, and a reminder that, with God, we can find hope even in the darkest hours.

Each chapter gently guides you through the various aspects of grief. We'll explore the complexities of our emotions and learn to view grief as a process that leads to personal and spiritual growth. Take each section at your own pace, allowing time to reflect, pray, and breathe. Whether you're just beginning this journey or have been walking it for some time, I hope these words bring comfort and remind you of God's closeness. My prayer is that you feel seen, held, and encouraged, knowing that there is hope, healing, and that God is with you every step of the way.

Please note that any names used in this book are fictional, and are intended to protect the privacy of those whose experiences have inspired these stories. The stories are drawn from a blend of real experiences, but any identifying details have been changed to honor confidentiality.

With all my heart,

Dr. NJ Domrufus, DNP, PMHNP-BC

Chapter 1: The Tapestry of Grief and Faith

Grief is more than a single, isolated feeling—it's a whole tapestry, woven from countless threads of memory, sorrow, joy, and love. When we lose someone we cherish, we don't just lose a person; we lose part of our identity, part of our world. Suddenly, we find ourselves living in a new reality, one that feels sharp-edged and unfamiliar. In those moments, grief becomes not just a feeling, but a journey that touches every part of who we are, calling us to make sense of a world that feels irreversibly altered.

And woven through this experience, if we allow it, is faith. Faith is the anchor in the storms of loss, the quiet, resilient strength that keeps us from drifting too far from ourselves. Faith doesn't take away the pain, but it offers us a safe harbor—a place to catch our breath, to gather our strength, and to remember that we're held, even in the darkest moments.

Understanding Grief as a Multifaceted Experience

Most of us think of grief as just feeling sad for a while—something that starts, happens, and eventually ends. But grief isn't that simple. It's a complicated journey that affects every part of us: our mind, body, heart, and soul. Grief can be messy, confusing, and very personal. Sometimes, there are even moments of unexpected happiness. Everyone's grief is different because it's shaped by the relationship they had with the person they lost and the love they still feel.

Imagine grief like a mosaic—a picture made up of many different pieces. Some of those pieces are sharp and painful, like sadness, anger, or regret. Other pieces are softer, filled with warm memories, love, or even moments that make you laugh. Together, all these pieces form a whole picture—a story of the connection you had, the loss you feel, and the memories that stay with you. And just like a mosaic, no two people's grief looks exactly the same.

When we understand that grief is made up of many layers and feelings, it helps us realize that it's okay to feel however we need to feel. Grief doesn't follow a set path, and it doesn't just "get better" in a straight line. Sometimes we feel a deep sadness, other times anger comes up, and sometimes we might feel nothing at all. And all of that is okay. Grieving isn't a sign of weakness or that we're not moving forward. It's proof of the love we still carry inside.

I once heard someone say, "Grief is love that has nowhere to go." That really stuck with me. The feelings of grief are just our hearts trying to make sense of losing someone we love, trying to figure out where all that love can go now. When we see grief as a mosaic, we can accept all of the different emotions we feel, knowing that each one is important to our healing. Grief is a way of showing that our love is still there—and that kind of love is always worth holding on to.

Faith: The Unseen Anchor in the Storms of Loss

Faith is like an unseen anchor that holds us steady when we face the storms of loss. It keeps us grounded in something bigger than ourselves, something that offers hope beyond what we can see. But what happens when that anchor isn't there? I remember talking to a client who had just lost his father—a sudden, unexpected loss that left him shattered. When I offered my condolences and said, "He's in a better place now," he looked at me with tired, empty eyes and quietly replied, "I don't believe in that." His words were raw and honest, cutting through any comforting assumptions I had. It made me realize how much harder grief must be without the hope that faith brings.

At that moment, I could feel the weight of what it must mean to grieve without believing in something beyond this life—without the hope that a loved one has found peace, or the comfort that there's a reunion waiting someday. It's one thing to grieve; it's another thing entirely to grieve without any hope, to feel like the love and memories are just suspended in emptiness, with nothing to hold onto.

As I watched that client wrestle with his pain, I felt a deep empathy for him. Grief, by itself, is a fierce storm. But grief without hope? That's a storm that feels endlessly dark, like being lost at sea with no direction or peace. Faith, for those who embrace it, becomes that unseen anchor, a reminder that love isn't limited to this life, that there's something more waiting beyond the horizon.

"And now, dear brothers, I want you to know what happens to a Christian when he dies so that when it happens, you will not be full of sorrow, as those are who have no hope." —1 Thessalonians 4:13 (TLB).

The Bible speaks to this when it says we shouldn't "grieve like those who have no hope". Now, that doesn't mean faith makes grief easy or takes away the pain. Grief will always be heavy, complicated, and deeply personal. But faith adds a thread of hope, a belief that our loved ones aren't just gone—they're held by something greater, something everlasting. Faith gives us a sense that our relationship with those we've lost doesn't end but shifts. It takes on a new form, one that allows us to carry them with us in a different way.

"Blessed are they that mourn: for they shall be comforted." —Matthew 5:4 (KJV).

Faith is the substance of things hoped for, the evidence of things not seen (Hebrews 11:1). It's about leaning into the word of a loving God who reminds us that we're held, even when we feel broken. The Word of God is alive, full of strength, and it has the power to lift us, encourage us, and guide us through any season of life. When we fill our minds and hearts with Scripture, we're allowing God's promises to come alive in us. We're building an unshakable faith that reminds us we are never alone, that we are loved, and that God is working all things together for our good. Faith may not always explain the "why"

5

behind our suffering, but it reminds us that we're part of a bigger story—one that has room for both our joy and our sorrow.

I think of faith like an anchor dropped deep into the ocean. The waves may be fierce, the winds may be relentless, but the anchor holds. Sometimes, we can't see or feel it; sometimes, we might even question if it's there at all. But faith is that steady pull, the unshakable certainty that even in the turmoil, there's something strong enough to hold us together.

For many of us, this anchor is found in prayer. In those quiet moments when we're honest with God—when we bring our questions, our anger, and our heartbreak without any filters. For others, faith is found in Scripture, in words that speak to our suffering and remind us that God is near. Those words become a lifeline, a reminder that God doesn't abandon us in our pain.

"The LORD is my solid rock, my fortress, my rescuer. My God is my rock— I take refuge in him!— he's my shield, my salvation's strength, my place of safety" Psalm 18:2 (CEB).

Faith also connects us to a community, to others who have walked through similar valleys of grief and found their way through. Their stories remind us that we're not the only ones. There's a kind of strength that comes from knowing we're part of something bigger, from sharing our experiences with others who "get it." And in that sharing, we find that we're not alone in the journey. Faith binds us together, even when everything else feels like it's falling apart.

A Journey, Not a Destination

Grief isn't something you just get over. It's not a finish line you cross or a destination you reach. It's a journey—sometimes winding, sometimes uphill, and always evolving. And as you walk this path, faith becomes more than just a solution; it becomes your companion. It's the steady presence that stands by you when you're in the valleys, and it's there to celebrate those precious glimpses of joy when they come.

I want to encourage you, as you move through these pages, to give yourself permission to feel every part of your journey. Grief isn't about being strong all the time. It's about letting yourself cry, laugh, ask the tough questions, and even be angry. It's about feeling it all—the full range of emotions—knowing that God is right there with you in every single moment. Faith doesn't demand perfection. It doesn't ask you to have it all together. It simply invites you to bring your whole, raw, honest self before God, just as you are.

Grief may never completely leave us, but it does change us. It stretches us, it deepens us, and in a mysterious way, it makes us more human. We carry the love of those we've lost with us—not in the same way, but in a way that reshapes us. And faith helps us see that this reshaping isn't a loss of who we are; it's an expansion. It's about becoming someone who understands both joy and sorrow on a deeper level. It's about being more genuine, more compassionate, and loving more fiercely than ever before.

My prayer is that this journey of grief and faith will lead you to new depths of understanding, compassion, and strength. May you find the courage in your faith, even when there are unanswered questions. And may you always know that God is walking right beside you, holding you steady, guiding you forward, and anchoring you in a love that is greater than any storm. Grief may be an ongoing process, but faith is the unchanging companion that walks with us, reminding us that even in our darkest times, we are never alone.

Chapter 2: Finding Comfort in Ancient Words

In the stillness that follows loss, grief can leave us feeling stuck—caught between what used to be and what lies ahead. In those moments, it can feel like words are meaningless, like nothing anyone could say could truly reach the ache in our hearts. But somehow, the timeless words of Scripture have a way of breaking through. They cross the barriers of time and enter into our pain, offering comfort—not with quick fixes, but with the promise of God's presence. A presence that walks with us through every valley, every shadow.

The beauty of Scripture is that it doesn't shy away from the reality of our suffering. It doesn't pretend that pain isn't real. Instead, it meets us there, in the rawness of our sorrow, and speaks to our hearts with a familiarity that brings unexpected comfort. In the words written by prophets, kings, and disciples, we find a deep understanding of what it means to be human. It's as if these verses already know what we're going through, as if they're waiting for us—ready to meet our pain and welcome it into a story that's far bigger than our moment of hurt. A story that reminds us that we are never alone, and that God's love is present, even in the darkest valleys.

Verses that Echo Through the Valley of Sorrow

The Bible is not merely a book of hope but also a book that understands the language of despair. It's this duality that makes Scripture such a powerful companion in times of grief. From the poetic lamentations of David to the raw questions of Job, these verses do not rush to conclusions or offer simple answers. Instead, they give voice to the depth of our pain and invite us to wrestle with it in God's presence.

"The Lord is close to the brokenhearted and saves those who are crushed in spirit."- Psalm 34:18 (NIV)

This verse speaks to the heart of grief. In the ancient words of Psalm 34:18, we find a profound statement of God's nearness—a promise that in the very moments we feel most abandoned, God draws closer. There's an intimacy in this verse, a whisper that assures us we are not lost in our sorrow but held within it.

The image is like that of a parent who sits beside a child in the dead of night, their presence a quiet comfort, a tangible reminder that they are not alone. When we are brokenhearted, God is not distant or indifferent. He doesn't stand apart from our suffering, but instead, He enters it with us. Psalm 34:18 gives us permission to grieve with the knowledge that we do so in the presence of One who cares deeply.

The Journey Through Despair

Job's story is one of the most powerful examples in the Bible about facing suffering. Job went through a lot—he lost his children, his job, his money, and even his health. He felt terrible, but he didn't pretend everything was okay. Job was very honest with God. He asked questions like, "Why did I not die when I was born?" (Job 3:11). Job's questions were raw and painful, showing us what true despair looks like.

The important part of Job's story is not that he got clear answers, but that he had the courage to ask the hard questions. Job's cries to God became a way for us to see that it's okay to ask our own questions when we're hurting. God is not upset by our pain. Instead, He listens to us, even when we don't understand why we're suffering. God meets us right there—in our confusion, in our sadness, and in our anger.

The story of Job shows us that God is not far away when we are in pain. He is close to us and wants to help us through it. Even when we don't get the answers we want, God is there, offering comfort and love. By being honest with God about our pain, like Job was, we can find a deeper connection with Him. It is in our hardest moments, when we bring our pain to God, that we discover He has been with us all along, ready to hold us and help us heal.

Walking Through the Valley

Psalm 23 is one of the most comforting passages in all of Scripture. It's a powerful reminder that we're never alone, even when life takes us through dark and challenging places. This psalm doesn't shy away from the difficult times; instead, it acknowledges them head-on and promises us God's presence right in the midst of them.

"Even though I walk through the valley of the shadow of death, I will fear no evil, for you are with me; your rod and your staff, they comfort me." - Psalm 23: 4 (ESV)

Notice, it doesn't say we avoid the valley—it says we walk through it. But here's the good news: we're not walking through it alone. The valley represents those tough seasons—the times when things aren't going the way we hoped, when we're feeling lost, discouraged, or afraid. But even in the middle of that darkness, our Shepherd is there. God is not a distant observer watching from above. No, He is right there, walking beside us, guiding us, comforting us, and giving us strength when we need it most. When you feel overwhelmed, remember that the Creator of the universe is holding your hand, leading you step by step.

Psalm 23 is God's promise that the pain you're experiencing is not forever. The valley is not where you'll end up—it's just part of your journey. You may walk through it, but you're not going to stay there. God is leading you to something better. He is the light in your darkness, and His rod and staff bring you both comfort and protection. They remind you that His love is greater than any fear, and His presence is stronger than any shadow. With Him, that valley becomes a journey of faith—a journey where every step brings you closer to God's amazing plan for your life. And when you come out on the other side, you'll look back and see that every moment in that valley made you stronger, more resilient, and more connected to your Heavenly Father.

Insights That Transform Pain

When we go through hard times, it's normal to ask questions—both about ourselves and about God. We wonder why we have to suffer and why a loving God would allow such pain. These are big questions that people have asked for a very long time, even in the Bible. The Bible doesn't give us simple answers, but it invites us to explore these questions. By thinking about them, we can understand both ourselves and God better.

In the Bible, many people struggled with these same questions. For example, in the book of Psalms, we see David asking God why he has to suffer. Instead of hiding his pain, David brought his honest questions to God. This teaches us that it's okay to ask hard questions. When we bring our doubts and pain to God, He listens and helps us grow.

Just like Jesus cried out when He was hurting, we can also share our pain with God. It's in these honest moments that we can grow closer to Him. When we are struggling, we have a choice: to turn away from God or to turn toward Him. If we choose to turn toward Him, we find that God meets us in our pain and helps us find strength we never knew we had. Hard times is not easy, but it can help us know God better and feel His love more deeply. It teaches us to depend on God and reminds us that we are never alone in our struggles. Our pain becomes a way for us to see how God works in our lives and brings us closer to Him, transforming our suffering into an experience of His grace and comfort.

Invitation to Intimacy with God

Sometimes, the hardest moments in our lives bring us closer to God. When we feel pain, it can be a chance to get to know God better. Pain takes away our defenses and makes us realize we need help. We can either turn away or choose to reach out to God, who is always ready to help us. When we choose to turn to Him, we find that God is closer to us than we could ever imagine, even in the middle of our deepest sadness.

In the Bible, there are many examples of people turning to God in their hardest moments. Jesus Himself showed us how to do this. When He was feeling very sad and scared in the garden of Gethsemane, He prayed to God the father, telling Him exactly how He felt.

"Then He said to them, 'My soul is deeply grieved, so that I am almost dying of sorrow. Stay here and stay awake and keep watch with Me'." - Matthew 26:38 (AMP)

This shows us that when we are hurting, God wants us to come to Him, to be honest, and to share our pain with Him. Nobody wants to suffer, and God doesn't want His children to be in pain. Just as Jesus turned to God when He was in pain, we can do the same. When we are honest with God about our pain, we can feel His love more deeply. We realize that He is always there, ready to help us through our hardest moments.

"The LORD is close to the brokenhearted; he rescues those whose spirits are crushed." - Psalm 34:18 (NLT)

God is near us when we are sad. He doesn't leave us alone in our pain. Instead, He comes closer to us, and it is often during our toughest times that we feel His love the most because we are leaning on Him completely. When we suffer, it can be a special chance to get to know God better. We learn about His compassion, His love, and His strength. When we reach out to God in our pain, He meets us with open arms, reminding us that we are never alone. God knows our pain, and He walks with us every step of the way.

"So be strong and courageous! Do not be afraid and do not panic before them. For the LORD your God will personally go ahead of you. He will neither fail you nor abandon you." - Deuteronomy 31:6 (NLT)

Path to Greater Compassion

Suffering not only draws us closer to God, but it also enlarges our capacity for compassion. When we endure loss, we gain a deeper understanding of the human condition—an understanding that cannot be learned from comfort alone. Our brokenness becomes the very thing that enables us to sit with others in their pain, not with empty platitudes but with empathy born of experience.

"Blessed [gratefully praised and adored] be the God and Father of our Lord Jesus Christ, the Father of mercies and the God of all comfort, who comforts and encourages us in every trouble so that we will be able to comfort and encourage those who are in any kind of trouble, with the comfort with which we ourselves are comforted by God."- 2 Corinthians 1:3-4 - (AMP).

Paul's words in 2 Corinthians 1:4 remind us that God comforts us so that we, in turn, can comfort others. This is the redemptive cycle of suffering: our pain becomes the very soil from which kindness and connection grow.

The Redemption of Suffering

At the core of our faith is a powerful truth: God is a God of redemption. He has this amazing ability to take what's broken, what seems hopeless, and turn it into something beautiful. No matter how painful the situation, nothing is beyond His reach. In Romans 8:28, we're reminded that *"in all things God works for the good of those who love him."* This verse did stated all things are good, or that we'll always understand why we're going through what we're going through. But it does promise that God is with us, right in the middle of our pain, and He's working—behind the scenes, weaving even our darkest moments into a greater story of grace, purpose, and hope.

The bible did not mention that God doesn't ignore our pain or pretend it's easy. It doesn't try to put a shiny bow on our grief. Instead, the word of God invites us to look at our pain through a different lens—to see it as part of a greater narrative. It's a story where every chapter matters, even the ones filled with heartache. It's a call to believe that our tears are not in vain, that our sorrow has the potential to be transformed. When we put our brokenness in the hands of a loving God, He has the power to take even the heaviest burdens and turn them into something meaningful and beautiful. It's a reminder that, no matter what we face, God's not finished with our story yet—He's still at work, bringing beauty from the ashes and turning our pain into purpose.

Finding Strength in Sacred Words

Scripture doesn't just speak to us—it sings to us. It reaches into our hearts in those moments of loss and reminds us of a hope that can lift us up. In those ancient words, we find a powerful truth: God doesn't abandon us in our sorrow. No, He meets us right there in the midst of our pain, and He transforms that grief into something that shows the depth of His love for us.

The beauty of Scripture lies in its honesty. It doesn't shy away from the messiness of life or the mystery of faith. It doesn't pretend that everything is perfect. When we walk through the valley of grief, these sacred words offer us more than just comfort. They offer us a new way of seeing our situation—a reminder that we are held by something bigger, something eternal, something that will never let us go. In the middle of our pain, we can find strength in God's Word, courage in His promises, and hope in the One who walks beside us every single step of the way.

Chapter 3: Mapping the Terrain of Grief

Grief is like trying to find your way through a huge, unknown wilderness—an unpredictable journey with steep hills, deep valleys, and winding paths that sometimes seem to lead nowhere. It's not about going in a straight line from start to finish; it's about learning the landscape, even when it feels confusing. We try to understand this unknown journey—not to make it sound easy or to pretend that everyone's journey is the same, but to see that while each person's grief is different, there are feelings that we all share. Grief is very personal, but it's also something that connects us all, and there's comfort in knowing that others have gone through this too.

Grief isn't a problem that we need to fix or something we can just get over. It's a journey—a process that takes us from feeling broken to finding healing, even if it's a bumpy road. Together, we'll look at the different parts of grief—not as a strict set of steps, but as a way to understand our feelings. We'll explore how faith can be part of this journey, how sadness and hope can exist together, and how prayer can guide us when we feel lost. Grief can be complicated, but we don't have to face it by ourselves. It's a human experience that connects us all and reminds us that, even in our darkest times, there is a way forward.

Navigating the Stages: A Guide to Understanding Emotional Landscapes

Grief is often described in different stages, but it's important to remember that these stages don't always happen in order, and we may revisit some of them multiple times. The stages of grief—denial, anger, bargaining, depression, and acceptance—represent common emotional experiences that many people go through as they navigate loss. Let's take a closer look at these stages and explore how we can recognize and navigate them.

1. Denial: The Numbness of Loss

Denial is often the first reaction to loss. It's the stage where we can't fully believe or accept what has happened. Denial acts as a protective shield, giving us time to process the shock of losing someone we love. You might find yourself thinking, "This can't be real," or "This isn't happening," or feeling disconnected from the reality of the loss.

> *Denial isn't a sign of weakness; it's the mind's way of giving us time to process what's happened.*

Allow yourself the time you need to come to terms with the loss. Denial can be a natural way for your mind to adjust to the overwhelming emotions. It's okay to take things slowly and to ask for support from those around you as you begin to face the reality of your grief.

2. Anger: The Frustration of Loss

Anger often comes when the reality of the loss starts to sink in. It's normal to feel angry at the situation, at the person who has died, at yourself, or even towards God. "Why did this happen?" and "How could this be allowed?" are questions that often come to the surface. You might feel that life is unfair or that you've been let down by others.

> *Anger is a powerful emotion that can help us feel a sense of control when everything seems uncertain.*

It is important to allow space for this anger, to acknowledge it without shame, and to remember that even anger can be a form of connection—a way of continuing to love what has been lost. Find healthy ways to express your anger. Talking with friends or family members, journaling, or even physical activities like exercise can help you release these feelings. Remember, it's okay to be angry—grief is a natural response to loss, and anger is part of that process.

3. Bargaining: The "What Ifs" and "If Onlys"

Bargaining is when we start to think about "what if" and "if only" scenarios. It's a reflection of our longing—a longing to have our loved ones back, to rewrite our story without the pain of loss. You might find yourself wishing you could go back in time or thinking of ways the loss could have been prevented. "If only I had done something differently" or "What if I had been there?"

Bargaining is a reflection of our longing—a longing to have our loved ones back, to rewrite our story without the pain of loss.

It's the mind's way of trying to regain a sense of control, even if it means making impossible deals. Recognize that bargaining is a way of coping with feelings of helplessness. It's natural to think about what could have been different, but try to be gentle with yourself and understand that the past cannot be changed. Lean on your faith or trusted support systems to help you move forward.

4. Depression: The Weight of Reality

Depression in grief isn't necessarily a clinical condition; it's a natural part of the grieving process. This stage can bring deep sadness, loneliness, and a sense of emptiness. The reality of loss sinks in. The numbness of denial fades, the questions of bargaining quiet down, and we are left with the raw, aching truth of what has happened. You might feel like withdrawing from others or losing interest in activities you once enjoyed. It is okay to feel this sadness—to cry, to mourn, to allow ourselves to fully experience the pain.

The sadness is deep because the love was deep.

During this depressive stage, it's important to remember that you don't have to go through it alone. Reaching out to family, friends, or a counselor can provide comfort and support. Allow yourself to feel the sadness without judgment. It's also helpful to find small activities that bring you moments of relief—like taking a walk, reading, or praying.

5. Acceptance: The Grace of Moving Forward

Acceptance doesn't mean that everything is okay or that the pain is gone. Instead, it means that you begin to accept the reality of the loss and start to learn how to live with it. This stage is about finding a new way of being—one where you carry the memory of your loved one while still moving forward in your life.

Acceptance is not an endpoint; it is a state of grace, a recognition that we can hold both grief and hope in our hearts simultaneously.

Acceptance takes time, and it's a gradual process. Give yourself grace as you adjust to this new reality. Seek out moments of joy and peace, no matter how small, and lean into your faith as you learn to rebuild. Acceptance doesn't mean "getting over" the loss; it means finding a way to carry it while also continuing to live.

Recognizing the Stages

It's important to understand that these stages aren't linear—you won't necessarily experience them in order, and you may revisit some stages several times. You might feel anger one day, acceptance the next, and then suddenly find yourself back in denial. That's normal, and it's part of the unpredictable nature of grief.

To recognize where you are in your grief journey, take time each day to check in with your emotions. Ask yourself how you're feeling and acknowledge those feelings without judgment. Remember, grief is a personal journey, and there's no right or wrong way to experience it.

By understanding the different stages and allowing yourself to move through them, you give yourself the space you need to heal. And through it all, your faith can be the steady presence that keeps you anchored, even when everything else feels uncertain.

Faith Intersections: Where Sorrow Meets Hope

Grief often brings us to a crossroads—a place where sorrow and hope meet. It's in these moments, when we feel most broken, that our hearts are most open to the whispers of faith. It's in the gentle reminders, the quiet assurances, that we realize we're not alone in our pain. Even though faith isn't a magic cure and it doesn't take away the sting of loss. But it does give us a foundation to lean on when everything else feels unsteady.

Think about a lighthouse standing strong in the middle of a storm. The waves may crash, the winds may roar, but the light never wavers. That's what faith is like when we're grieving. It's the steady light that guides us, even when we can't see where we're going. Faith points us toward hope, reminding us that our loved ones aren't lost to us forever—that there is a promise of reunion, that death is not the end but a doorway to something greater.

Faith allows us to sit with our sorrow, knowing that it's not meaningless. It gives us the courage to face the darkness because we know God is right there with us. In those moments of deepest pain, God's presence is closest. It's in these intersections of sorrow and hope that we discover a depth of strength we didn't know we had—a strength that comes from knowing we are held by something greater than ourselves. We are held by a God who sees our tears, who knows our pain, and who promises that joy will come again. So even when you're walking through the valley, remember that the light of faith is still shining, leading you forward one step at a time.

Chapter 4: Marking the Milestones

Grief is not something that happens just once; it has a way of revisiting us, especially on anniversaries and special dates that hold deep significance. These milestones—birthdays, anniversaries, holidays—carry echoes of the love we've lost and can bring waves of emotion crashing down on us. And yet, these moments also hold the potential for profound healing and remembrance. They remind us of what mattered most and offer us a chance to honor that love in meaningful ways.

In this chapter, we'll explore how to navigate these milestones with compassion, courage, and grace. We'll look at strategies for coping with the emotions that come with these reminders and reimagine rituals that can help us celebrate the lives of those we've lost. Grief isn't about letting go; it's about finding new ways to carry the love with us—ways that enrich our lives instead of weighing us down.

Strategies for Navigating the Echoes of the Past

Anniversaries and special dates can feel like emotional landmines—reminders of what once was, of moments shared, and of the love that still lingers. And the thing is, it's okay to feel everything that comes with those reminders. The goal isn't to avoid the pain, but rather to navigate it with tenderness toward ourselves.

1. Acknowledge the Day

The first step in navigating these difficult days is to acknowledge them. Pretending these dates are just like any other day can make the pain even heavier. Instead, allow yourself to recognize the significance of the day. It's okay to feel the sadness, the longing, and even the anger that comes with it. Give yourself permission to feel whatever comes up without judgment. Grief is not something that can be neatly packaged away; it's part of who we are, and acknowledging it is an act of courage.

A conversation with Sarah, a woman who lost her father five years ago. She shared how, on the anniversary of his passing, she used to pretend the day was just like any other, hoping that if she ignored it, the pain would be less intense. But it wasn't. Eventually, she decided to acknowledge the day instead. She now lights a candle in her father's honor, allowing herself to feel whatever comes. Some years, she laughs at the memories; other years, she cries. But each time, she feels a sense of connection to her father that brings her comfort.

2. Plan Ahead

One of the best ways to navigate anniversaries and reminders is to plan ahead. Planning ahead is a way of creating a good distraction. Think about what might make the day a little more bearable for you. Would it help to spend time with loved ones, or would you rather have some quiet time alone to reflect? Would visiting a favorite place, cooking a special meal, or listening to a particular song bring comfort? Planning ahead gives you some control over the day and creates space for remembrance that feels meaningful. Rather than spending the day overwhelmed by sadness, use the time to plan and create something. Directing that energy into making something meaningful or building connections with loved ones can transform the day into one of purpose rather than sorrow.

Mark lost his wife unexpectedly. On the anniversary of her passing, he plans a day of reflection. He visits their favorite hiking spot—a place where they shared countless joyful moments—and brings along a picnic filled with her favorite foods. He said that the first year, it felt impossible to face the day, but planning these small rituals has helped him find a way to honor her and create moments of peace amidst the grief.

---

3. Create Space for Grief and Joy

Grief and joy can coexist—even on the most difficult days. You can honor the sadness of loss while celebrating the beauty of the memories you hold. On an anniversary, you might choose to light a candle in remembrance and then spend time doing something that brings you joy—like taking a walk in nature, cooking a favorite dish, or creating art. Creating space for both grief and joy allows you to honor the fullness of your emotions and the depth of your love.

Emma shared how she copes with her mother's birthday each year. She starts the day by baking her mother's favorite cake, a recipe passed down through generations. Later, she takes her children to the park where they release balloons in her mother's memory. The day is filled with both tears and laughter—a bittersweet mix that honors the beautiful complexity of their relationship.

---

4. Reach Out for Support

Grief can be incredibly isolating, especially on significant dates. Reaching out to friends or family members who understand your loss can be a powerful way to find comfort. Let others know that you may need extra support on these days—whether that means a phone call, a visit, or simply someone to sit with you in silence. Sharing your grief with those who care about you can lighten the burden and remind you that you're not alone in this journey.

On the anniversary of his brother's death, he will always make sure to call their mutual best friend. They'll share stories, laugh about the good times, and sometimes even cry. He says those calls remind him that his brother's life mattered not just to him, but to everyone who knew him, and it makes the weight of the day a little lighter.

Rituals Reimagined: Creating New Traditions to Honor Memory

Rituals are an essential part of how we process grief and keep the memory of our loved ones alive. When someone we love passes away, the rituals and traditions we once shared can feel empty or painful. But reimagining these rituals can provide a new way to honor their memory and keep their spirit present in our lives.

1. Honoring Through Acts of Kindness

One beautiful way to reimagine rituals is to honor your loved one through acts of kindness. Consider creating a new tradition where, on significant dates, you perform an act of kindness in their memory. It could be something small, like buying coffee for a stranger, volunteering at a local charity, or writing a letter to someone who needs encouragement. These acts of kindness become a way to channel your love and keep your loved one's spirit alive in the world.

Maria, who lost her grandfather—a man who was known for his generous heart. On his birthday each year, she performs an act of kindness in his memory. One year, she bought groceries for a struggling family; another year, she volunteered at a local shelter. She told me that these acts of kindness help her feel close to her grandfather, as if his spirit is still at work in the world through her.

---

2. Memory Jars and Storytelling

Another meaningful way to honor your loved one is by creating a memory jar. On anniversaries or special dates, gather friends or family members and invite them to write down a favorite memory on a piece of paper. Place these memories in a jar, and over time, watch the jar fill with stories, moments, and reflections that celebrate the life of the person you lost. Storytelling is a powerful way to keep their memory alive—it allows us to share the joy they brought to our lives, and it connects us with others who also carry pieces of their story.

The Thompson family started a memory jar after their son, James, passed away. Each year on his birthday, they invite friends and family to contribute a memory to the jar. They sit together, read the

*memories aloud, and share laughter
and tears. Over the years, the jar has
become a treasured collection of James's
spirit—filled with stories that remind
them of the joy he brought into their
lives.*

---

3. Create a Space for Reflection

Sometimes the best way to honor a loved one is to create a physical space for reflection. This could be a small garden, a memorial bench, or even a dedicated corner in your home with photos, candles, and mementos. This space becomes a sanctuary where you can go to feel close to your loved one, to reflect on your journey, and to find peace in the presence of their memory. Creating such a space can be a comforting way to incorporate their memory into your daily life.

---

*Struggling to find a way to honor her
mother, Anita created a small garden
filled with her mother's favorite
flowers. Every morning, she spends a
few minutes there—watering the
plants, sipping her coffee, and
reflecting on her mother's life. This
space has become a sacred part of her
day, a place where she feels her
mother's presence most deeply.*

---

4. New Traditions for Old Holidays

Holidays can be particularly challenging after a loss because they carry the weight of traditions shared with those we love. Reimagining these holidays can help ease the pain and create new ways to celebrate. If you used to cook a special meal together, consider inviting friends or family to cook it with you in honor of your loved one. Or, if certain traditions feel too painful, create entirely new ones that reflect your current reality while still paying tribute to the past. The goal isn't to erase what was, but to find ways to adapt and honor the love that remains.

After losing her sister, she found it impossible to continue their usual Christmas traditions. She created a new one—each year, she invites friends over for a holiday dinner and asks them to bring a dish that reminds them of someone they love. It has become a beautiful way to honor not only her sister's memory but also the memories of others, turning a painful holiday into a celebration of love and connection.

Moving Forward with Grace

Milestones and anniversaries will always hold a special place in the journey of grief. They are moments that remind us of what we have lost, but they are also opportunities to reflect on the love that remains. By finding ways to navigate these echoes of the past and reimagining rituals that bring meaning to our memories, we allow ourselves to move forward with grace. May we find strength in these moments, may we honor the past while embracing the present, and may we walk forward, knowing that love never truly leaves us—it simply changes form.

Chapter 5: The Communion of Healing

Grief can be one of the loneliest experiences—it makes us feel like we're drifting all by ourselves in a sea of sorrow. But let me tell you something: grief is also deeply communal. There's a healing power that comes when we let others into our journey, when we share our stories, our tears, our laughter, and our prayers. You see, God never meant for us to walk through these valleys alone. He designed us for connection, for community, for the kind of relationships that lift us up when we feel like we can't go on.

In this chapter, we're going to explore what I like to call the communion of healing. We'll talk about how prayer serves as a refuge, a safe place where we can pour out our hearts to God and find peace. We'll also see how the people around us—our friends, our family, our church community—can be God's hands and feet, bringing us comfort when we need it most. And we'll talk about how to build those networks of support, the kind that hold us up during our darkest hours.

Grief isn't something we're meant to face on our own. It's a journey that we're called to walk together, hand in hand, hearts connected by shared understanding and love. When we open ourselves up to others, when we allow people to come alongside us, we discover that there's strength in numbers. We realize that our burdens become lighter when they're shared, and our joy becomes greater when it's celebrated together. So let's lean into the communion of healing. Let's find comfort in prayer, strength in community, and hope in the knowledge that we are never alone. God is with us, and He's placed people around us to help us along the way.

Prayer as a Refuge

When words fail us, when we don't know where to turn, prayer becomes our refuge. It's that sacred place where we can lay it all out— every fear, every doubt, every tear. You don't need to have it all figured out to come to God. He doesn't ask for perfection or polished words. He just asks that you come, just as you are—raw, broken, vulnerable.

In those moments of deep grief, when it feels like the weight of the world is pressing down on you, prayer is your lifeline. It's the way we connect with the One who holds the universe in His hands, and yet cares deeply about every single detail of our lives. When we pray, we're not just speaking into the void; we're entering into a conversation with the Almighty, the One who sees our pain, who hears our cries, and who promises to be with us through it all.

Prayer is where we find solace when everything else feels shaky. It's where we find the peace that surpasses all understanding, the kind of peace that doesn't come from our circumstances but from knowing that God is with us. So when the world feels heavy, when your heart feels overwhelmed, remember—you have a refuge. You have a God who is listening, who is near, and who is ready to meet you right where you are. Just come to Him, and let His presence be the anchor that holds you steady.

1. Honest Conversations

Prayer is not about reciting perfect words or pretending that everything is okay. It is about having an honest conversation with God, even if that means bringing our anger, our confusion, and our pain to Him. Sometimes, we might find ourselves saying, "God, I don't understand why this happened," or "I'm angry that You allowed this." These words are not blasphemous; they are a genuine expression of our hearts. And God, in His infinite compassion, can handle our honesty. I remember a conversation with Laura, a woman who lost her son to a sudden illness. She told me how, in the weeks after his death, she couldn't bring herself to pray the way she used to.

Instead, she found herself sitting in silence, sometimes weeping, sometimes just asking, "Why?" Over time, she realized that those moments of silence—those moments of raw, honest emotion—were her prayers. They were the deepest conversations she had ever had with God. Prayer, she learned, wasn't about having the right words; it was about showing up, even in her brokenness.

---

2. Finding Solace in Scripture

In times of grief, there's nothing quite like the words of Scripture to bring healing to our wounded hearts. You see, God's Word has a way of meeting us right where we are—especially when we're hurting. The Psalms, in particular, are filled with the raw, honest emotions of those who cried out to God in their distress.

"So do not fear, for I am with you; do not be dismayed, for I am your God. I will strengthen you and help you; I will uphold you with my righteous right hand." - Isaiah 41:10 (NIV).

Isn't this a beautiful promise? These words remind us that God is near, that He is right there with us, ready to strengthen and uphold us, and that we are never alone. When we pray, we can draw on these verses, letting them anchor us in the midst of our pain. It's like God is whispering, "I see you, I'm with you, and I'm holding you." For so many people, repeating these verses becomes a way of meditating on God's truth—a way of steadying their hearts when the waves of grief seem too much to bear. It's not about finding an answer to the "why" of our suffering, but about finding comfort in the knowledge that we have a God who walks with us through every single moment.

God's Word is like a healing balm, soothing our hearts when they feel shattered. It's a reminder that even in the midst of our darkest valleys, we are held by the One who loves us most. So when grief feels overwhelming, turn to Scripture. Let those ancient words wash over you, let them remind you of God's goodness, and know that He's right there, walking beside you, every step of the way.

The Role of Community in the Mosaic of Healing

While prayer provides an intimate connection with the God, community offers us the opportunity to connect with others who understand our pain. Grief can feel like a heavy burden to carry alone, but when we share it with others, the weight becomes just a little more bearable. The people around us—our family, friends, church members—become part of the mosaic of our healing, each one contributing a piece to help us rebuild what has been broken.

1. The Power of Presence

Sometimes, the most powerful thing we can do for someone in grief is simply to show up. No words of wisdom, no advice—just being there.

Think of John, a man who lost his wife after a long, courageous battle with cancer. He told me about his friend, who came over every day after her death. His friend didn't try to fill the silence with empty reassurances. He just sat on the porch with John, shared a cup of coffee, and watched the sun dip below the horizon. "It was his presence that helped me through those days," John said. "He didn't try to fix anything; he just sat with me. And that was enough."

This is the power of presence. It's the willingness to be there with someone in their pain, not to solve it, but to share it. Grief isn't a

31

problem to be solved, and it's not something we can take away from each other. But we can bear witness to each other's pain, and in doing so, we help lighten the load just a little bit.

Some people, when faced with grief, feel the urge to withdraw from everyone around them. They shut themselves up, avoiding visitors or guests, thinking that solitude will help them process their emotions. While there is value in having moments of quiet reflection, isolating completely can often make the burden of grief even heavier. Allowing others to be present, even if it's just for a short time, helps share the weight of grief and makes the journey a little more bearable. Grieving in a healthy way involves letting people in—letting them sit with you, listen to you, or just be with you. It's in those shared moments that real healing begins. It's not about having the right words; it's about having the right heart. Being there, without pretense or pressure, is often the most meaningful thing we can do.

When we show up for others, we remind them they're not alone. The simple act of presence tells someone, "I see you, and I'm here for you." In a world that often pushes us to fix things and offer solutions, there's something truly powerful about just sitting together, embracing the silence, and knowing that being there is enough.

2. Sharing Stories

One of the most healing aspects of community is the ability to share our stories. When we share our grief, we give others permission to share theirs as well. It creates a space where we can be vulnerable, where we can say, "I'm struggling," and know that we will be met with understanding rather than judgment.

I think of a grief support group I attended years ago. There was a woman named Mandy who had lost her sister, and she was struggling to find her way through the pain. As she shared her story, another woman in the

group, Maria, reached over and took
her hand. Maria had lost her brother
the year before, and as she listened to
Mandy, she nodded, tears streaming
down her face. "I know exactly how you
feel," Maria said. "And you're not
alone." In that moment, Mandy found a
connection that brought her comfort—
someone who truly understood her
pain. That is the gift of community: the
ability to say, "Me too."

Building Networks of Support: Practical Steps for Engaging Faith Communities

Faith communities can be a powerful source of support during times of grief. They offer us a sense of belonging, a reminder that we are part of something bigger than ourselves. But engaging with these communities can feel daunting when we are in the midst of deep sorrow. Here are some practical steps for building networks of support within your faith community.

1. Reach Out and Be Honest About Your Needs

One of the hardest things to do when we're grieving is to ask for help. We often tell ourselves that we don't want to burden others, or we believe that we should be strong enough to handle things on our own. But the truth is, none of us are meant to go through grief in isolation. We need each other. Reaching out to your community—especially your faith community—and being open about what you need can unlock support you never knew was available.

The thing is, grief doesn't come with a rulebook. There's no "right way" to move forward. But what we do know, from research and from human experience, is that connection matters. People want to help, but they often don't know how. By being honest about what we need—

whether it's a listening ear, help with daily tasks, or simply someone to sit beside us—we invite others to be part of our journey. And in doing so, we not only receive the support we need, but we also allow others the opportunity to show up in meaningful ways. It's not a sign of weakness to ask for help; it's a sign of being human. And it's often the first step toward genuine healing.

I remember an experience I had in the Costco parking lot. I was pushing my shopping cart, loaded with two or three packs of water and toiletries, while also carrying my baby. A middle-aged gentleman happened to be passing by, and he approached me, offering to help. I instinctively turned him down, but he insisted. Again, I politely declined, telling him I was fine. Then he made a profound statement: "Why can't you let me help you?" His words struck me because here I was, visibly struggling, yet still refusing help. It dawned on me how often we have people who are willing to lend a hand, but we push them away, trying to put up a facade of strength even when we're struggling inside.

This experience taught me a valuable lesson: when you're in pain or need help, reaching out is important, but it's equally important to accept the help that's offered. Whether it's family, friends, or your church community, allowing others to help you doesn't make you weak—it makes you human. Accepting help is an act of courage, a way of acknowledging that you don't have to do it all alone, and that there is strength in community.

2. Join or Start a Support Group

Many faith communities offer support groups for those who are grieving. If your church has such a group, consider joining it. These groups provide a safe space where you can share your story, listen to others, and find comfort in knowing that you're not alone. But what if your community doesn't have a support group? You could be the one to start it. It doesn't have to be anything formal—sometimes, the most meaningful connections happen in a small circle of people willing to be vulnerable together.

I think of David, who decided to start a small grief group at his church after losing his mother. He felt an overwhelming sense of isolation in his grief, and he wanted to create a space where others could come together. What began with just three people grew into a close-knit community that gathered every week to share, pray, and support each other. David once told me, "It's not just about my healing anymore; it's about helping others heal too."

That's the power of support groups. They create an environment where healing becomes a shared experience, where one person's courage to speak can inspire another to do the same. It's a ripple effect—when one person opens up, it makes space for others to share their stories. Whether you're joining a group or starting one, the impact goes beyond just you. It's about building a community of care, where everyone's pain matters and everyone's journey is respected.

The truth is, grief is not something we're supposed to navigate alone. It's not a solitary path, but a journey best traveled in the company of those who understand. A support group isn't about fixing each other's pain—it's about sitting in the messiness of it together, about knowing that even in your lowest moments, there are people who will sit beside you, hold space for your story, and remind you that hope is still there, even if you can't see it right now.

3. Participate in Corporate Worship

There's something uniquely powerful about coming together in worship, especially during times of grief. Singing hymns, praying alongside others, and listening to messages of hope can offer a profound sense of comfort and connection. Even when it feels like the hardest thing to do, participating in corporate worship is a way of reminding yourself that you're not alone—you're part of a community that cares about you, that is ready to support you, and that walks with you through the valleys.

I think of Mary, who lost her father and, for a time, stopped attending church. The thought of being around people who seemed happy was just too painful when her heart felt so broken. But one Sunday, she made the decision to go back. As the congregation began to sing, tears filled her eyes, and she felt something shift within her. "I realized that I wasn't alone," she said. "Everyone around me was lifting me up, even if they didn't know it. It was the first time I felt a glimmer of hope again."

That's the power of worship. It reminds us that even when we're struggling, even when we feel like we can't find our way, we're not on this journey by ourselves. Grief is not a journey we're meant to walk alone. It's a path that we navigate together, carried by our prayers and surrounded by people who love us. Prayer gives us a way to connect with God—to pour out our hearts, to be raw and honest, and to find refuge in His presence. Community gives us a way to connect with each other—to share our stories, to sit in the silence, to laugh, to cry, and to lift each other up when the burden feels too heavy.

In the communion of healing, we find that while the pain may not disappear, we are never truly alone. We find strength, comfort, and hope—not in the absence of grief, but in the presence of love, in the presence of others who are willing to stand with us. Worship becomes an act of solidarity, a reminder that there's light, even when the valley seems darkest. It's about knowing that, together, we can lift our voices, lift each other, and in doing so, lift ourselves closer to hope.

Chapter 6: The Alchemy of Grief

Grief has the power to transform us in ways we might never have imagined. It is a journey through the shadows, a personal odyssey that forces us to confront the depths of our own vulnerability and strength. But grief, when faced with courage and openness, can become a catalyst for transformation. It can take the weight of our sorrow and turn it into something meaningful—something that honors the love we lost and shapes the person we become. This chapter is about the alchemy of grief—how we can transform loss into legacy, find growth in the shadow of loss, and envision a future full of purpose and hope.

The Personal Odyssey: Growth in the Shadow of Loss

Grief is not a straight path; it's like a winding road that takes us through moments of feeling sad, angry, or lost. Everyone's journey through grief is different, but even in the hardest times, we can grow and become stronger. It's not always big changes; sometimes it's small steps forward that help us heal.

But within the darkness, there is also growth.

Imagine someone who has lost someone they love very much. At first, the pain feels like it takes over everything. It can be hard to think or even breathe. But slowly, small steps happen. Maybe it's getting out of bed in the morning, even when it feels too hard. Maybe it's going outside to feel the sun or talking to a friend. These little acts are brave, and they help us move forward, even when it feels impossible. Grief makes us stronger in ways we might not expect. It shows us that we can rise up, even when we feel broken. It helps us see the little bits of light in our lives, even if they don't last long.

Grief teaches us to be kind to ourselves and reminds us that growing doesn't mean forgetting the person we lost—it means learning how to carry the love and memories with us in a new way.

Growing after a loss doesn't mean going back to who we were before. It means becoming someone new—someone who knows both happiness and sadness deeply. It means living fully, even though we know life can be fragile. It means loving deeply, even though we understand that loss is part of life. And in this way, grief helps us become more understanding, more caring, and more alive.

Grief as a Catalyst for Change

Grief changes us. It takes away the idea that we have complete control, and it makes us face the truth that life is sometimes unpredictable and hard. But within this challenge, there is also the chance to grow. Grief, when we face it with an open heart, can help us change in powerful ways.

Think about someone who has lost a loved one—a parent, a partner, or a close friend. At first, they may feel overwhelmed by sadness, anger, and confusion. They may wonder if they will ever feel okay again. But slowly, as they go through the grief, they start to notice other things too—like what really matters in life and how precious their relationships are.

Grief is like fire—it can hurt, but it can also purify.

Grief can teach us to live with purpose, to appreciate every moment, and to love without holding back. It can push us to make changes in our lives—chasing our dreams, fixing broken friendships, or letting go of the fears that stop us from living fully. It can lead us to reevaluate our priorities, to recognize that life is too short to be lived in half measures.

One of the biggest ways' grief helps us grow is by giving us a new purpose. Many people who have experienced a deep loss find themselves wanting to honor their loved one's memory in special ways. They might start a foundation, volunteer for a cause that mattered to their loved one, or simply try to live in a way that reflects the values of the person they lost. In this way, grief becomes more than just pain— a catalyst that pushes us to become the best version of ourselves, to live a life that honors both the love and the loss.

Envisioning a Future: Redefining Purpose with Faith

When we are in the depths of grief, it can be hard to imagine a future that is anything but empty. The idea of moving forward feels impossible, like a betrayal of the love we lost. But envisioning a future does not mean forgetting—it means finding a way to carry that love with us, to allow it to shape the path ahead.

Faith plays a powerful role in helping us redefine our purpose after loss. It gives us a sense of hope, a belief that there is more to this life than what we can see and touch. It reminds us that, even in our darkest moments, we are not alone.

God walks with us through the valley of sorrow, and He has a plan for our lives, even when we cannot see it.

Envisioning a future means allowing ourselves to dream again, to imagine what life could be, even in the absence of the person we lost. It means finding new ways to bring joy into our lives, to connect with others, to make a difference in the world. It means recognizing that our loved one would want us to live fully, to find happiness, to continue growing and evolving.

For some, redefining purpose might mean taking on a new role— becoming a mentor, a volunteer, a caretaker. For others, it might mean pursuing a passion they once set aside, or simply finding joy in the small moments of everyday life. One example of this is someone who, after losing a spouse, decides to dedicate their time to helping others who are grieving. They become a source of comfort and support for those who are walking the same path, using their own experience to help others find their way. In doing so, they find a new sense of purpose—one that honors their spouse's memory and brings meaning to their own life.

> *Redefining purpose with faith is not about forgetting the past—it is about building a future that honors the love we carry with us.*

Another example is a person who, after losing a child, decides to pursue a passion they had long neglected. They take up painting, writing, or gardening—something that brings them a sense of peace and fulfillment. Through this creative expression, they find a way to honor their child's memory, to keep their spirit alive in the work of their hands.

Redefining purpose is about trusting that, even in the midst of our pain, there is hope. It is about believing that God has a plan for our lives, and that He can take the broken pieces of our hearts and create something beautiful. Whatever form it takes, redefining purpose is about choosing to live with intention, to honor the love we lost by creating a life that is rich and meaningful.

The Importance of Grieving Well: Embracing Health and Letting Go of Guilt

Grieving well is essential to our healing. It means allowing ourselves to fully experience the range of emotions that come with loss—sadness, anger, confusion, and even moments of peace. Grieving well is about giving ourselves permission to feel, without judgment or shame. It means recognizing that there is no "right" way to grieve, and that the journey is different for everyone.

A crucial aspect of grieving well is letting go of guilt. Guilt can complicate grief, making it heavier and more difficult to bear. We may find ourselves feeling guilty for not doing enough for our loved one, for things left unsaid, or even for moments when we feel a glimmer of happiness. But guilt does not serve us in our healing journey. It keeps us stuck in the past, unable to move forward.

To grieve well, we must release the burden of guilt and embrace self-compassion.

We must remind ourselves that we did the best we could with the knowledge and resources we had at the time. We must allow ourselves to find moments of joy without feeling that we are betraying our loved one. Grieving well is about honoring the love we shared, while also allowing ourselves to heal and grow.

Grief is a journey that takes us through the darkest valleys, but it is also a journey that can lead us to the most profound transformations. It is a journey of growth, of healing, of finding purpose in the midst of pain. The alchemy of grief is not about turning sorrow into joy, but about finding a way to live fully, even with the weight of our loss. It is about allowing the love we lost to shape the person we become, to inspire us to live with intention, to create a legacy that honors their memory.

As you move forward on your own journey, remember that growth takes time. Be gentle with yourself. Allow yourself to feel the pain, but also allow yourself to dream, to hope, to envision a future that is full of meaning and purpose. Grief may change us, but it does not have to define us. With faith, with courage, with love, we can transform our loss into a legacy that will endure, long after the tears have dried.

Chapter 7: A Continuum of Hope

Grief is a journey that demands courage—the courage to feel, the courage to be vulnerable, and the courage to keep showing up. I want you to remember that grief is not a destination. It is not something you "get over" or "move past." Grief is a continuum—a path you walk, a companion that will always be with you in some form. But grief is also a continuum of hope, a reminder that love endures, that transformation is possible, and that the deepest pain can give way to profound beauty.

Reflecting on the Journey: Key Takeaways

Grief strips us down to our most vulnerable selves. It is raw, it is painful, and it is deeply personal. But in that vulnerability lies the opportunity for transformation. Throughout this book, we've explored the alchemy of grief—the way it can reshape us, strengthen us, and lead us to a deeper understanding of our own hearts. As we reflect on this journey, I want you to hold onto a few key takeaways, the ones that I hope will stay with you in the days, months, and years to come.

First, give yourself permission to feel everything. Grief is messy, unpredictable, and nonlinear. There will be days when you feel like you're making progress, and days when the weight of your loss feels just as heavy as it did in the beginning. That's okay. There is no right way to grieve—there is only your way, and it is enough. Allow yourself to feel the sadness, the anger, the confusion, and even the moments of peace. Honor every emotion as it comes, without judgment or shame.

Second, be kind to yourself. Grief is not a journey that comes with a timeline or a set of instructions. It is not something you can rush through or check off a list. Healing takes time, and it looks different for everyone. Be gentle with yourself as you navigate the ups and downs. Talk to yourself as you would talk to a friend—with compassion, patience, and love. Remind yourself that you are doing the best you can, and that is more than enough.

Third, lean into your community. We are not meant to grieve alone. The people around you—your family, your friends, your faith community—are there to hold you up when the weight of grief feels too heavy to bear. Let them be there for you. Let them see your vulnerability. There is so much power in allowing others to witness our pain. It creates connection, it fosters empathy, and it reminds us that we are not alone.

The importance of not grieving alone cannot be overstated. When we isolate ourselves in our grief, we amplify the weight of our sorrow, and it becomes an unbearable burden. The beauty of community support— whether from family, friends, faith communities, or support groups— is that it allows us to share that burden. It reminds us that we do not have to carry the weight alone, that there are others willing to hold us up when we feel like we might collapse.

The Role of Family and Friends: Sharing the Weight of Grief

Family and friends are often the first line of support when we face a profound loss. They are the people who know us best, who understand the nuances of our relationships, and who can offer a sense of familiarity and comfort when everything else feels foreign and frightening. Opening up to them, sharing our memories, expressing our emotions—all of these acts create a space of love and acceptance where the weight of grief is shared, rather than carried alone.

One woman who lost her partner found solace in her family gatherings, where they shared stories, looked at old photographs, and laughed together. These moments did not erase her pain, but they lightened the load. They reminded her that she was not alone, and that her partner's memory would always be kept alive through the love of those who knew him.

Leaning into family and friends does not mean that we need to have all the right words or that we need to be strong for others. It means showing up as we are—broken, vulnerable, and real. It means allowing others to hold us when we cannot hold ourselves.

The Importance of Support Groups: Finding Strength in Shared Experience

Support groups provide a unique kind of comfort—one that comes from knowing that the people around you truly understand what you are going through. Unlike family and friends, who may not have experienced a similar loss, support groups are filled with people who are walking their own path of grief. This shared experience creates a deep sense of understanding, empathy, and validation, which is crucial for healing.

Support groups can be found in various forms—locally, online, through social media—and they have become an invaluable resource for many. Take for instance one man grieving the loss of his mother attending a support group specifically for adults who had lost a parent. Hearing others share their stories might make him feel less alone. It will validat his emotions, and possibly provided him with practical coping strategies for his difficult days. He might also find some level of comfort and perhaps a sense of purpose—a desire to help others who were just beginning their journey.

Support groups offer these kinds of experiences. I have seen many of my clients improve in a matter of months. There is something profoundly healing about being in a space where you do not have to explain yourself—where your pain is understood without words. They remind us that we are not alone, that there is strength in shared vulnerability, and that healing is possible when we come together.

Faith Communities and Spiritual Support: Anchoring Ourselves in Belief

For those whose faith provides a framework for understanding loss, engaging with a faith community can be a powerful source of support. Whether it is attending services, participating in prayer groups, or

45

connecting with a spiritual leader, these communities offer both emotional and spiritual support. They help us anchor ourselves in the belief that there is something greater than our pain, something that holds us even when we feel like we are falling apart.

A grieving father found solace in his church community, which rallied around him and his family. They brought meals, offered prayers, and simply sat with him in his grief. The sense of belonging he felt—the spiritual guidance and the unwavering support—helped him find hope and trust in a higher plan. In his darkest moments, he was reminded that he was not alone, and that his faith could be a source of strength and comfort.

Faith communities remind us that we are not meant to walk this journey alone. They offer a space where our pain is seen, where our questions are heard, and where our spirits are nurtured. They provide a place where we can find meaning, even in the midst of our suffering, and where we can be reminded of the promise of hope that is found in our faith.

Allowing Others to Witness Your Pain: The Courage of Vulnerability

Grief often makes us feel exposed and vulnerable. It can be incredibly difficult to let others see us in our pain, to allow them to witness the depth of our sorrow. But there is so much power in allowing others to witness our grief. When we let people in, when we share our pain, we create a space where true healing can happen—both for ourselves and for those who stand beside us.

After losing her best friend, one woman found herself retreating from those around her. She didn't want to burden anyone with her pain, and she felt as though no one could truly understand. Eventually, though, she decided to reach out to a close friend and share her true feelings. To her surprise, her friend responded with compassion, and they spent hours talking about her loss. That conversation marked the beginning of her journey to healing. It helped her feel seen and understood, and it reminded her that vulnerability is not weakness—it is strength.

Allowing others to witness our pain takes courage. It means letting go of the fear of being judged, and it means trusting that the people who love us are willing to hold space for our grief. It is in these moments of shared vulnerability that we find the deepest connections, the kind that remind us that we are not alone and that we are loved, even in our brokenness.

Seeking Counseling and Taking Care of Mental Health: Finding Your Way Forward

In addition to leaning on family, friends, support groups, and faith communities, it is also important to recognize the value of professional support. Grief can be overwhelming, and sometimes, despite the love and support of those around us, we need additional help to navigate the depth of our emotions. Seeking counseling or therapy can be an incredibly important step in the healing process.

Counseling provides a safe and non-judgmental space to explore the complexities of grief.

Grief therapy allows you to express your emotions freely, to work through feelings of guilt or anger, and to develop coping strategies that can help you move forward. For some, medication may also be a helpful tool in managing the symptoms of grief, particularly if it has led to depression or anxiety. There is no shame in seeking the help you need to take care of your mental health—it is an act of strength, an acknowledgment that you deserve to heal.

Taking care of your mental health while grieving is about keeping your head above the water. It is about recognizing that you cannot pour from an empty cup, and that in order to heal, you must take care of yourself—mind, body, and spirit. It is about giving yourself permission to seek the support you need, to lean on the resources available to you, and to trust that healing is a journey, not a destination. It may take time, and it may require different forms of support along the way, but with each step forward, you are honoring both your own well-being and the love you have for the one you lost.

Walking Beside God: Embracing an Eternal Partnership

Grief can feel like a journey we take all by ourselves, but it doesn't have to be that way. In our sadness, God invites us to remember that we are not alone. Walking with God means having Him as our partner, guiding us through the hardest times and celebrating with us in the good moments. It means trusting that God is holding us, even when it feels like everything is falling apart.

God doesn't need us to have it all together. He wants us to come to Him just as we are—hurt, confused, and honest.

Life isn't always easy, and we all have times of heartache and pain. But remember, you don't have to face those struggles by yourself. Imagine you are walking along a path that is rough and uncertain. There are moments when you trip and fall, and times when the weight of your grief feels impossible to carry. Then, in those hardest moments, you feel a presence beside you—a hand reaching out, a gentle voice reminding you that you are not alone. That is what it means to walk with God. He is there, not to take away our pain, but to walk with us through it, giving us strength when we have none left, and helping us when we're too tired to take another step.

God doesn't promise that we won't face tough times, but He does promise that we won't face them alone. And the amazing thing is that when we lean on Him, He gives us the strength we need, even when we feel like we can't go on. It's about being honest with God, sharing our pain, our questions, and our fears with Him. There's something deeply comforting about knowing that our journey is part of something bigger—an eternal story where every tear is seen, every hurt is held, and every loss is known.

*Even when the path is tough, we are
not abandoned. God knows our pain
deeply, and He promises to guide us
through it with His love and care.*

Walking with God means trusting His promises, even when we don't fully understand them. It means believing that there is hope beyond the sadness, that there is light beyond the darkness, and that the love we carry is forever. In this journey of grief, God is not far away—He is our partner, our guide, and our comfort. As we lean on Him, we find that while grief may be part of our story, it is not the end. With God by our side, we can keep moving forward with hope, knowing we are never truly alone. There may be tears, but there is also the promise of joy. There may be sadness, but there is also the promise of peace. And with God walking beside us, we know that brighter days are still ahead.

Benedictions: Prayers for the Road Ahead

As we come to the close of this journey, let's take a moment to rest, reflect, and breathe deeply. In those quiet moments of prayer, we find the strength we need to face whatever lies ahead. These prayers are like gentle whispers from heaven, wrapping us in comfort, guiding us with love, and filling our hearts with hope for tomorrow. No matter how heavy the days may feel or how uncertain the road may seem, these blessings remind us that God's peace goes with us, His love surrounds us, and His strength holds us steady.

*You've got this, and more importantly,
God's got you.*

Benedictions are blessings that carry us forward—not as people who have it all figured out, but as people who are deeply loved by God. Let them remind you that the journey of grief is not one you must walk by yourself. You have a loving Father who is walking right beside you, understanding your pain, and leading you toward a future filled with hope. Remember, the God who is walking with you today will be with you tomorrow and every day after that. Life's road may have twists and turns, but you're not traveling it alone.

"Do not be afraid or discouraged, for the LORD will personally go ahead of you. He will be with you; he will neither fail you nor abandon you."
Deuteronomy 31:8 (NLT).

Take these prayers with you as you move forward. Let them be your anchor on days when your heart feels heavy, and your spirit feels weary. You have a faithful companion in God—one who blesses every step you take, who knows the weight of your sorrow, and who promises that brighter days are ahead. Step by step, prayer by prayer, you are not alone. And as you continue on this journey, may you find that God's love is not just with you—it is ahead of you, lighting the path, bringing you peace, and leading you to a place of healing and joy.

Jesus told her, "I am the one who raises the dead and gives them life again. Anyone who believes in me, even though he dies like anyone else, shall live again. He is given eternal life for believing in me and shall never perish. Do you believe this, Martha?" — John 11:25-26 (TLB).

Prayer Points and Affirmations

Prayer for Comfort in Times of Sorrow

Father, I thank You for Your promise to be close to the brokenhearted. In my moments of deepest sorrow, I ask that You wrap me in Your love and bring comfort to my spirit. I trust that You are my refuge, and that in You, I can find rest. (Psalm 34:18 – *"The Lord is close to the brokenhearted and saves those who are crushed in spirit."*)

Declaration of Trust in God's Presence

I declare that I am not alone in my grief. The Lord is with me, walking beside me through every valley. His presence is my peace, and His love sustains me through every difficult moment, in Jesus name. Amen. (Isaiah 41:10 – *"So do not fear, for I am with you; do not be dismayed, for I am your God. I will strengthen you and help you; I will uphold you with my righteous right hund."*)

Prayer for Strength to Move Forward

Heavenly Father, grant me the strength to face each new day, even when it feels impossible. I pray for Your courage to help me take one step at a time, trusting that You are guiding me and that my future holds hope. (Philippians 4:13 – *"I can do all things through Christ who strengthens me."*)

Affirmation of God's Faithfulness

I affirm that God is faithful, and His promises are true. He has plans for my future—plans to give me hope, not harm. Even in my pain, I will hold on to His Word, believing that He is working all things together for my good, in Jesus name. Amen. (Jeremiah 29:11 – *"For I know the plans I have for you," declares the Lord, "plans to prosper you and not to harm you, plans to give you hope and a future."*)

Prayer for Peace Beyond Understanding

Lord Jesus, You promised a peace that surpasses all understanding. I ask for that peace now. In the chaos of grief, let Your peace settle over my heart and mind, calming my fears and soothing my pain, in Jesus name. Amen. (Philippians 4:7 – *"And the peace of God, which transcends all understanding, will guard your hearts and your minds in Christ Jesus."*)

Declaration of Hope in God's Eternal Love

I declare that my hope is found in the love of God. His love never fails, and His compassion never ends. I will not allow grief to overshadow the truth that I am deeply loved and cared for by my Heavenly Father. (Lamentations 3:22-23 – *"Because of the Lord's great love we are not consumed, for His compassions never fail. They are new every morning; great is Your faithfulness.*")

Prayer for Healing and Restoration

Father God, I bring my brokenness before You. I ask for Your healing touch upon my heart and my soul. Restore to me the joy that grief has taken, and help me to see glimpses of Your goodness even in the midst of my pain, in Jesus name. Amen. (Psalm 147:3 – "*He heals the brokenhearted and binds up their wounds.*")

Affirmation of God's Comforting Presence

I affirm that God's presence is my comfort. Though I may walk through the darkest valleys, I will fear no evil, for He is with me. His rod and His staff, they comfort me. (Psalm 23:4 – "*Even though I walk through the darkest valley, I will fear no evil, for You are with me; Your rod and Your staff, they comfort me.*")

Prayer for Community and Support

Lord, I thank You for the community You have surrounded me with. I ask that You use them as vessels of Your love and comfort in my life. Help me to be open to their support, and let me find strength in the relationships You have blessed me with, in Jesus name. Amen. (Ecclesiastes 4:9-10 – "*Two are better than one, because they have a good return for their labor: If either of them falls down, one can help the other up.*")

Declaration of a Future Filled with Hope

I declare that grief is not the end of my story. With God, there is always hope. I believe that He is guiding me to a future filled with His promises, His love, and His peace. I will walk forward in faith, knowing that brighter days are ahead, in Jesus name. Amen. (Romans 15:13 – "*May the God of hope fill you with all joy and peace as you trust in Him, so that you may overflow with hope by the power of the Holy Spirit.*")

Appendices

Tools for the Journey

Grief isn't a straight path, and it's not something you have to do by
yourself. Sometimes it can feel confusing and hard, like you're lost
and don't know which way to go. But the most important thing to
remember is that you don't have to do it alone. In this part of the book,
I've shared tools, resources, and ways to get support to help you on
your journey of healing. These are not magic solutions that will make
everything better right away. They are like stepping stones to help you
when things feel too heavy, and to remind you that you are not alone.
Grief is something that all people go through, and it helps to know that
there are many ways to find hope, comfort, and understanding.
Remember, you are never alone, and there are always people and
resources out there to support you.

Resources and Support Networks

As you navigate the complexities of grief, having tools and resources
readily available can make all the difference. Sometimes, the weight of
sorrow is simply too much to carry by ourselves. Whether you need
someone to talk to, practical coping strategies, or a community that
understands what you are going through, these resources can be
invaluable. Below are several types of support available to you:

- Support Groups: These are communities of people who have
  experienced similar losses. Support groups provide a safe space
  where you can share your experiences without judgment and be
  understood by others who truly know what you are feeling.
  Many groups meet in person, while others meet online or
  through social media platforms. Whether you connect locally
  or virtually, support groups remind us that we are not alone in
  our grief.

- Therapeutic Tools: Consider journaling, art therapy, or
  physical activities like yoga and walking to support your
  mental and emotional health. Writing down your feelings or
  engaging in creative expression can help release the emotions

that words alone cannot capture. Physical activity is also a powerful tool in managing grief, as it allows your body to process the emotions held within it.

- Faith-Based Resources: If your faith is an important aspect of your life, lean into your faith community. Attend services, participate in prayer groups, or seek the counsel of a spiritual leader who can provide both emotional and spiritual support. Many find solace in knowing that their faith offers a foundation of hope and meaning, even when life feels uncertain.

- Counseling and Therapy: Professional counseling can be incredibly beneficial during times of loss. A counselor can help you explore your emotions, offer coping strategies, and provide a space where you can talk freely about your grief. Therapy is not about "fixing" your pain; it is about allowing yourself to be held in your grief and finding a way forward with support.

These tools are meant to help you feel supported, seen, and understood. Remember that reaching out for help is an act of courage, and no one is meant to grieve alone.

A Curated List of Grief Counseling Services

Grief counseling can provide you with the individualized support you need as you navigate your loss. It offers a space where your grief is validated, where your emotions are met with compassion, and where you can work through the many layers of your experience.

Here is a curated list of grief counseling services to help guide you in finding the support that is right for you:

1. National Grief Support Hotline: This hotline provides immediate support for those experiencing grief, as well as information on local grief resources and counseling options. Available 24/7, it can be an essential point of contact when you need someone to listen.

2. Local Grief Counseling Services: Many hospitals and community centers offer grief counseling or referrals to

professional counselors specializing in grief and loss. Reaching out to a nearby hospital or mental health clinic can help you find local resources that may not be widely advertised.

3. Faith-Based Counseling: If your faith is an important part of your healing journey, consider seeking grief counseling through your place of worship. Many churches, synagogues, mosques, and other religious institutions provide pastoral counseling for those experiencing loss.

4. Online Counseling Platforms: Online therapy is a valuable resource, particularly for those who may not have access to in-person services. Platforms such as BetterHelp and Talkspace provide licensed therapists who specialize in grief, allowing you to connect with support from the comfort of your home.

5. Specialized Grief Counseling Centers: Some counseling centers specialize specifically in grief and trauma. They offer a wide range of services, including individual counseling, group therapy, and workshops designed to help you process your grief in a safe and supportive environment.

There is no one-size-fits-all approach to grief counseling. Find the service that speaks to your needs, and know that seeking help is not a sign of weakness—it is an act of strength, a declaration that you deserve support, and that you are worthy of healing.

Recommended Readings: Books for Deeper Understanding

Books have always been a source of comfort, insight, and connection, especially when it comes to understanding grief. Below, you will find a curated list of recommended readings—books that offer different perspectives on loss, hope, and the journey toward healing.

1. "The Year of Magical Thinking" by Joan Didion: A profound memoir that chronicles Didion's experience of grief after the sudden death of her husband. It is a raw, honest exploration of the disorienting nature of loss, and it offers readers a poignant insight into the complexities of grief.

2. "Option B: Facing Adversity, Building Resilience, and Finding Joy" by Sheryl Sandberg and Adam Grant: This book is a powerful combination of personal storytelling and practical advice. Written after the sudden loss of her husband, Sheryl Sandberg shares her journey of finding resilience and joy after unimaginable loss. It also provides valuable insights into how we can support others in their grief.

3. "Grieving Mindfully: A Compassionate and Spiritual Guide to Coping with Loss" by Sameet M. Kumar: This book blends mindfulness practices with insights into grief, offering a compassionate guide to navigating loss. It provides practical tools to help readers sit with their grief in a way that fosters healing and understanding.

4. "When Breath Becomes Air" by Paul Kalanithi: Written by a neurosurgeon who was diagnosed with terminal cancer, this memoir is an eloquent reflection on life, death, and what gives our existence meaning. It offers readers a poignant reminder of the beauty and fragility of life, and it is a deeply moving meditation on loss.

5. "Tear Soup: A Recipe for Healing After Loss" by Pat Schwiebert and Chuck DeKlyen: A gentle and beautifully illustrated book that offers a metaphorical approach to grief. It is a comforting resource for both adults and children, helping readers understand that grieving takes time and that everyone grieves in their own way.

6. "It's OK That You're Not OK: Meeting Grief and Loss in a Culture That Doesn't Understand" by Megan Devine: This book challenges the cultural narrative that grief should be "fixed" or "overcome." Megan Devine writes from both personal and professional experience, offering a compassionate guide for those grieving and those who wish to support them.

These books offer different perspectives on grief, healing, and the human experience. They are not answers—they are invitations to explore, to feel, and to find comfort in knowing that others have walked similar paths and have found their way forward.

As you continue on your journey, remember that grief is a process that takes time, patience, and compassion. There is no right or wrong way to grieve—there is only your way. Lean on the tools and resources available to you, reach out to those who understand, and trust that there is hope on the horizon. You are not alone in this journey. You are part of a continuum of love, connection, and transformation. And most importantly, you are worthy of healing, of joy, and of a future full of hope.

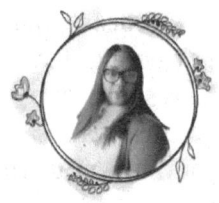

About the Author: A Glimpse into the Life of the Storyteller

Dr. NJ Domrufus is a storyteller, a compassionate listener, and a fierce advocate for healing. As a psychiatric mental health provider and a devoted Christian, her life's work has been dedicated to walking with others through their darkest moments and helping them find the light of hope. NJ's journey as both a mental health professional and a believer in the power of grace has allowed her to weave together the threads of faith, resilience, and human connection in every aspect of her work.

Growing up in a close-knit community, NJ learned early on the value of empathy and the strength that comes from vulnerability. She witnessed firsthand the power of coming together in times of need, and these experiences laid the foundation for her career in mental health. With a deep understanding of the human spirit and an unwavering belief in the transformative power of faith, NJ has spent years guiding individuals and families through the complexities of grief, trauma, and mental wellness.

Her professional journey has been shaped by her own encounters with grief and loss—experiences that have taught her that the path to healing is rarely straightforward but always worth pursuing. It is this personal understanding that has made her approach to mental health both deeply empathetic and profoundly effective. She believes that grief is not something to be conquered but rather a journey to be embraced, and she approaches every client with the conviction that healing is possible, even in the face of unimaginable pain.

When NJ isn't working with her clients, reading, or writing, she finds solace in her faith, her family, and the simple joys of life. Whether it's spending time with her loved ones, engaging in community outreach, or finding inspiration in the beauty of nature, she believes in the importance of nurturing the soul and finding moments of grace in the everyday. Her love for storytelling comes from a desire to connect, to uplift, and to remind others that they are not alone—no matter how heavy their burden may feel.

Navigating Grief with God: Finding Hope After Loss is more than just a book; it is NJ's heartfelt offering to those who are grieving. It is a testament to her belief that, even in our darkest moments, there is light to be found, love to be shared, and hope to be embraced. Through her words, NJ invites readers to join her on a journey of faith, healing, and transformation—a journey that is both deeply personal and universally human.

NJ's life is a reflection of the themes within this book: the courage to face our pain, the willingness to be vulnerable, and the faith that there is always hope on the horizon. She hopes that, through her writing, she can be a companion to those who are grieving—a voice that whispers, "You are not alone, and there is still beauty ahead."

More Books by NJ Domrufus

◊ Quiet the Food Noise: *Finding Faith and Freedom with Food*

◊ Guarding Your Soul Gates: *Protecting Your Heart and Mind as a Believer*

◊ Decline the Offer: *Rejecting Negative Whispers with God's Truth*

◊ The Discovery (Children's book story for ages 7 to 10 years of age)

◊ The Beatitudes Book Series (Children's book story series for ages 4 to 9 years of age)

◊ Heart & Soul Stories Series (Children's book story series for ages 4 to 9 years of age)

◊ How Doctors Take Care of You: A Visit to Dr. Kind's Clinic (Children's book story for ages 4 to 9 years of age)

◊ Brave Like David: *Facing Giants with Kindness* (Coloring Book)

◊ Strength for Today: *30 Days of Faith and Peace for Anxious and Heavy Hearts*

◊ Anchored in His Love: *Daily Meditation for Women* (a 5-Minute Daily Meditation for Women, designed to help you connect with God in a meaningful way, even on the busiest of days, featuring scripture, reflections, and inspiration to deepen faith.)

Look for these titles in stores and online soon!